I. Introduction:

In 2004 the Federal Trade Commission brought legal action retrospectively challenging the 2000 acquisition of Highland Park Hospital (HPH) by the Evanston Northwest Healthcare (ENH) hospital system, which prior to the merger had consisted of Evanston Hospital and Glenbrook Hospital. All three hospitals are in or near Evanston, Illinois. As discussed in Haas-Wilson & Garmon (2010), there is strong evidence that prices at the merging hospitals increased following the merger.[1] Balan & Garmon (2008) discuss FTC Complaint Counsel's interpretation of this price increase, and the alternative interpretation of Respondent's Counsel.

Respondent's Counsel claimed that the merger caused clinical quality at Highland Park Hospital to improve in several important ways.[2] The main purpose of this paper is to describe the analyses that we performed in response to those claims. Our study deals with clinical quality, as it has been defined by the Institute of Medicine and the World Health Organization, and not with hospital amenities. Some of our analyses relied on confidential data provided by the merging parties, and so cannot be reported here. However, the central component of our evaluation used publicly available quality measures and data, which can be reported (see Romano and Mutter (2004) for a detailed description of the variety of available measures of clinical quality). We find little evidence that the merger improved quality at Highland Park Hospital.

A secondary purpose of the paper is to lay out the conceptual framework that we believe should be applied in evaluating clinical quality claims in hospital merger cases, both retrospective and prospective. We discuss the basis for our prior belief that hospital mergers do not on average improve hospital quality, but are nevertheless likely enough to do so that substantial case-specific investigation is usually warranted. We also discuss the most likely sources of quality improvement, and ways to evaluate them.

II. Data, Quality Measures, and Empirical Methodology:

A. Data.

Our data source is the Illinois Department of Public Health (IDPH) Universal Dataset. This data set contains all inpatient discharges from nonfederal acute care hospitals in Illinois from 1998-2003. It contains information on the demographic characteristics of each patient, as well as ICD-9-CM (International Classification of Diseases, 9th Revision, Clinical Modification) diagnosis and procedure codes that describe the clinical condition of each patient and what procedures were performed. In preparation for trial, we also analyzed specialty-specific patient outcomes data from the National Registry of Myocardial Infarction, the Society for Thoracic Surgeons, and the National Perinatal Information Center, as well as patient satisfaction and experience data from the vendor Press Ganey. Hospitals voluntarily submit their data to these organizations and programs, and then receive benchmarking reports describing their performance in comparison with other facilities. The merging parties were required to provide these reports for review and analysis, and they were used in the first author's testimony, but they belong to the merging parties and therefore are not available to report here.

B. Quality Measures.

The primary quality measures analyzed in this paper come from Version 2.1 of the Inpatient Quality Indicators (IQIs) and the Patient Safety Indicators (PSIs) developed by the Agency for Healthcare Research and Quality (AHRQ). These indicators of health care quality make use of hospital inpatient administrative data such as the IDPH data, and focus principally on short-term patient outcomes. The IQIs reflect quality of care inside hospitals, including inpatient mortality for medical conditions and surgical procedures, and the PSIs focus on potentially avoidable

3

complications and iatrogenic events. To implement these measures, we ran the data obtained from the IDPH through a commercial "grouper" software program that used each patient's demographic information, diagnosis codes, and procedure codes to assign that patient to an "All Patient Refined Diagnosis Related Group" (APR-DRG) and to a Risk of Mortality (ROM) subclass. We then fed these APR-DRGs and ROMs, along with other elements from the IDPH dataset, into AHRQ's publicly-available Quality Indicator software for SAS to generate risk-adjusted outcomes measures. IQI risk-adjustment incorporates age, gender, age-gender interactions, circumstances of admission (i.e., transfer from another hospital), and APR-DRGs with ROM subclasses. PSI risk-adjustment incorporates age, gender, age-gender interactions, circumstances of admission, base DRGs (i.e., aggregated across comorbidity/complication levels), and AHRQ-defined comorbidities.[3]

The other quality measures that we used were developed by the Joint Commission on Accreditation of Healthcare Organizations, now known as The Joint Commission (TJC). TJC is the largest accrediting organization for acute care hospitals in the US; its accreditation review process includes a broad array of Core Measures that hospitals are required to collect and report. TJC maintains measures of risk-adjusted mortality for heart attack patients, neonatal mortality, and obstetric trauma. We purchased these measures, which are now publicly available on Medicare's HospitalCompare website but were not at the time, from a leading vendor (Iameter).

All of the analyses described in this paper involve patient outcomes. This is an appropriate focus, as outcomes are of ultimate interest to patients, their families, and policy-makers. However, data limitations make it difficult to judge a hospital solely on its outcomes. This is partly because hospitals often have a relatively small number of patients of a given type, which makes outcomes a noisy measure of quality; and partly because there are many outcomes that cannot be measured at all with available data, such as post-hospitalization mortality, quality of life, and functional status. For this reason, hospital quality researchers also use "structural" quality measures, which focus on whether organizations have the human resources and technical infrastructure to provide high-quality care, and "process" measures, which focus on the specific diagnostic and therapeutic services that organizations provide. At trial, the first author discussed several of these measures, but we do not discuss them here as they mostly relied on proprietary data obtained from the merging parties. For this reason, the results reported below are confined to outcomes measures from AHRQ and TJC, which represented the core of our analysis.

C. Empirical Methodology.

Our empirical methodology involves a series of difference-in-differences analyses of risk-adjusted mortality and complication rates for a number of clinical conditions. We evaluate whether the changes in these rates at the merged hospitals were different than the average change at a set of control hospitals. Changes in the control group rates serve as a counterfactual proxy for what the changes would have been at the merging hospitals absent the merger.

The virtue of difference-in-differences analysis is that confounding factors that do not vary over time (i.e., hospital fixed effects) are "differenced out." If the case mix of each hospital's patients did not change from year to year, then any differences in patient severity of illness would also be differenced out, and there would be no problem using raw mortality and complication rates in the analysis. But patient mix can change over time, particularly following a merger that may alter referral practices in the community, leading to differential changes in hospitals' case mixes. For this reason, we prefer to evaluate risk-adjusted mortality and complication rates, which are interpreted as the rate that a hospital would have had if its patients were of average severity. Even with the risk-adjustment, we recognize that some confounding is likely to persist due to omitted clinical factors.

The disadvantage of using risk-adjusted rather than raw rates is that risk-adjusted rates depend to some extent on hospitals' reporting practices. That is, when assigning diagnosis and procedure codes to patients, hospital coders rely upon physician documentation combined with their own professional experience and judgment.[4] Changes in these coding practices over time may confound the difference-in-differences exercise. However, these coding practices seem less likely to change differentially over time (after a merger) than patient severity, which is why we emphasize risk-adjusted rates while also reporting raw rates.

Following Haas-Wilson & Garmon (this issue), we performed our analysis using four different control groups. The first group consisted of all non-federal general acute care hospitals in the Chicago Primary Metropolitan Statistical Area (PMSA). Using hospitals in the Chicago area as controls offers the advantage of adjusting for unmeasured cost or environmental factors that may affect changes in hospital quality at the local level (e.g., percentage of residents without health insurance, county/state support for uncompensated care, Medicaid payment rates, local quality improvement or public reporting programs, state regulations regarding physician or hospital licensure), but it may underestimate the impact of the merger because some control hospitals may be close enough to be affected the merger, and may respond by reducing quality. The other three control groups[5] consisted of subsets of the Chicago PMSA hospitals that arguably were particularly similar to the hospitals in the ENH system. Since the other three control groups generated very similar results, we only report results using the first group.

The merger occurred in early 2000. We omit 2000 as a transition year, as any merger-induced changes would take some time to be implemented. We define the pre-merger period as

1998-1999, and the post-merger period as 2001-2003. Our primary concern is with changes in clinical quality at HPH, as it is at HPH that Respondent's Counsel claimed the merger improved quality. However, it is also possible that the merger could have had effects on clinical quality at Evanston Hospital and/or Glenbrook Hospital, as resources may have been diverted from Evanston or Glenbrook to Highland Park in such a way that Highland Park's gain was Evanston's or Glenbrook's loss. This effect is most likely to be present for cardiac services because ENH started a new cardiac surgery and interventional cardiology program at HPH, and the resources for that program were drawn largely from Evanston and Glenbrook. To simplify the presentation, we report only analyses on HPH and Evanston Hospital, but these results are not materially affected by adding Glenbrook Hospital.

We define our difference-in-differences estimator $\beta = \Delta p_{enh} - \Delta p_{control}$. Under the assumption of i.i.d. random sampling from a binomial distribution, the standard error of β is the denominator of the expression below. Therefore the following is (approximately) distributed standard normal under the null hypothesis that quality at ENH did not change relative to the control group:

$$Z = \frac{\left(p_{enh}^{post} - p_{enh}^{pre}\right) - \left(p_{control}^{post} - p_{control}^{pre}\right)}{\sqrt{\dfrac{p_{enh}^{post}\left(1-p_{enh}^{post}\right)}{N_{enh}^{post}} + \dfrac{p_{enh}^{pre}\left(1-p_{enh}^{pre}\right)}{N_{enh}^{pre}} + \dfrac{p_{control}^{post}\left(1-p_{control}^{post}\right)}{N_{control}^{post}} + \dfrac{p_{control}^{pre}\left(1-p_{control}^{pre}\right)}{N_{control}^{pre}}}},$$

where p represents the probability of the adverse outcome (death or complication) and N represents the number of patients.

III. Results:

The analyses that we performed were chosen in response to specific quality claims made by Respondent's Counsel. In this section, we discuss those claims, how we selected quality measures for testing them, and the results of the tests. As described above, we calculate pre- vs. post-merger absolute (percentage point) differences at the treatment hospitals, and then calculate the difference between those differences and the absolute differences at the control hospitals. We report both risk-adjusted and raw rate results, which are similar in most cases.

A. Cardiac Surgery and Interventional Cardiology.

After the merger, ENH established cardiac surgery and interventional cardiology programs at HPH, so that coronary artery bypass graft (CABG) surgery and percutaneous coronary intervention (PCI) procedures began to be performed there. Since there was no such program at HPH before the merger, no pre- vs. post-merger comparison is possible. But it is possible that the establishment of the program at HPH had an adverse impact on Evanston Hospital, as resources may have been diverted to support the new program at HPH.[6] To test this hypothesis, we analyzed the AHRQ Inpatient Quality Indicators for CABG and PCI mortality at Evanston Hospital. Results are reported in Table 1.

For CABG, the control hospitals experienced a 0.80% absolute reduction in risk-adjusted mortality, and EH experienced a 0.56% increase, for a difference-in-differences of 1.37%. For PCI, the decrease at the control hospitals was 0.11% and the increase at EH was 0.54%, for a difference-in-differences of 0.65%. Both of these estimates are in the direction of a quality reduction, although neither is statistically significant. In both cases, the effects are smaller (but in the same direction) for the raw rates than for the risk-adjusted rates.

B. Advantages of Teaching Hospitals.

There is evidence that teaching hospitals on average outperform non-teaching hospitals in caring for patients with a variety of conditions, including acute myocardial infarction (AMI, or heart attack), inpatient congestive heart failure (CHF), pneumonia, and stroke.[7] Respondent's Counsel claimed that the merger allowed HPH to realize the advantages of a teaching hospital.[8] Based on publicly available data, the first author argued that neither EH nor HPH met the definition of a teaching hospital, as defined in most prior studies (i.e., membership in the Council of Teaching Hospitals or at least 0.10-0.27 residents per bed). Nevertheless, we tested the claim by analyzing the AHRQ Inpatient Quality Indicators for those four conditions as well as the corresponding TJC indicator for AMI. Results are reported in Table 2.

According to the IQI measure, risk-adjusted AMI mortality at the control hospitals decreased by 1.88%, and increased at HPH by 0.34%, for a difference-in-differences of 2.22%. This finding suggests a decrease in quality at HPH, but is not statistically significant. However, for this measure there is an unusually large divergence between the risk-adjusted result and the raw difference-in-differences of -3.21% (also not statistically significant). Both the risk-adjusted and raw rates show a large and statistically significant decrease in quality at EH, difference-in-differences of 4.46% and 3.33%, respectively.

According to the TJC measure, risk-adjusted AMI mortality decreased by 1.52% at the control hospitals (compared to 1.88% according to the IQI measure), and decreased by 5.01% at HPH (compared to an increase of 0.34% according to the IQI measure), for a non-significant difference-in-differences of -3.48%. Similarly, the difference-in-differences at Evanston is -0.59%, as compared to an increase of 4.46% for the IQI measure. These differences may be partially explained by differences in risk-adjustment, and also by the exclusion of patients who were transferred in from other hospitals (as well as out-transfers) from the TJC measure; by contrast, the AHRQ measure only excludes out-transfers, because it is not known whether they survived the acute hospital stay. However, the discrepancy is large enough to cause us to suspect that there may have been a coding error in the commercial software that we used to group the APR-DRGs, in the AHRQ IQI software, or in the software used by Iameter to calculate the TJC measures.

CHF mortality improved non-significantly at both HPH (risk-adjusted difference-in-differences of -1.60%) and EH (-0.19%) after the merger. Risk-adjusted and raw pneumonia mortality and stroke mortality deteriorated non-significantly at HPH (risk-adjusted difference-in-differences of 0.30% for pneumonia and 2.42% for stroke). There was a large and statistically significant deterioration in risk adjusted pneumonia (3.14%) and stroke (4.94%) mortality at Evanston Hospital.

C. Nursing-Sensitive Indicators.

Another claim made by Respondent's Counsel was that the merger improved nursing care at HPH.[9] We evaluate this claim by examining Patient Safety Indicators that are known to be sensitive to the quality of nursing care, and that reflect concepts endorsed by the National Quality Forum (NQF) as voluntary consensus standards for nursing-sensitive care.[10] These include Decubitis Ulcers (pressure sores), Failure to Rescue (death among surgical patients with potentially serious but treatable in-hospital complications), Selected Infections Due to Medical Care, and Post-Operative Hip Fracture. Results are reported in Table 3.

HPH experienced slight post-merger deterioration for Post-Operative Hip Fracture (difference-in-differences in risk-adjusted rates of 0.10%), and improvements in the other three indicators (a statistically significant -0.76% for Decubitis Ulcer and non-significant -2.74% for Failure to Rescue and -0.01% for Selected Infections Due to Medical Care). However, for Decubitis Ulcer and Failure to Rescue, the raw differences-in-differences are much smaller in magnitude and in the case of Failure to Rescue it is of the opposite sign. The results for EH are mixed, with several nursing-sensitive PSIs showing statistically significant improvements.

D. Obstetrics.

Another quality claim made by the Respondent's Counsel was that the merger had improved obstetric care at HPH.[11] We evaluate this claim by examining the three PSIs that relate to obstetrics: Birth Trauma, Obstetric Trauma (Vaginal with Instrument), and Obstetric Trauma (Vaginal without Instrument). We also examine all three of the TJC obstetrics measures: Obstetric Trauma,[12] Neonatal Mortality, and Vaginal Birth after Caesarian (VBAC). Note that VBAC is not considered to be a quality measure in the traditional sense, but it reflects whether a hospital is capable of providing patient-centered care to women who have had prior cesarean deliveries. Results are reported in Table 4.

For the risk-adjusted obstetric PSI measures, results at HPH were unfavorable, with statistically significant deteriorations of 0.33% for Birth Trauma and 1.28% for Obstetric Trauma (Vaginal without Instrument), and a non-significant deterioration of 3.76% for Obstetric Trauma (Vaginal with Instrument). EH deteriorated on all three obstetric indicators, and the deterioration was statistically significant for Birth Trauma and Obstetric Trauma, (Vaginal with Instrument).

For the risk-adjusted TJC measures, HPH had a non-significant difference-in-differences of 0.12% for Neonatal Mortality, and a statistically significant -1.14% difference-in-differences for Obstetric Trauma. EH had statistically significant difference-in-differences of 0.32% for Neonatal Mortality and -1.08% for Obstetric Trauma.

IV. Interpretation of Results:

As can be seen in the tables, the standard errors on the Highland Park Hospital differences-in-differences estimates are generally quite large, so in many instances where the point estimate indicates a relative deterioration, substantial improvement cannot be ruled out. However, although we did not attempt a formal statistical test of whether quality improved "overall" across all the quality measures, our results taken together suggest that an overall improvement at HPH is unlikely, and that a large overall improvement is very unlikely.[13] This conclusion is reinforced by the fact that, as discussed below, the relevant literature does not support a prior belief that hospital mergers are likely to improve quality.

Our results must be interpreted with caution. The statistical significance of some findings may be overstated because we did not account for heterogeneity among control hospitals. We also cannot exclude the possibility of endogeneity; a decision to merge may reflect hospital managers' inside knowledge of emerging trends in quality, such that the experience of control hospitals may not represent what would have happened at the merging hospitals absent the merger.

V. Conceptual Framework:

A. Priors.

Since the ENH/HPH case was retrospective, our primary evidence came from our difference-in-differences analyses, which we used to directly measure the effect of the merger on clinical quality. However, the strength of the direct evidence required to reach a conclusion regarding the effect of a particular merger depends on one's prior beliefs regarding hospital mergers in general. These priors matter less when the direct evidence is strong, but absent completely persuasive direct evidence they still affect the posterior estimate of the merger effect. For this reason, we briefly review the relevant research that informs our prior belief that on average hospital mergers do not substantially improve clinical quality.

On balance, the empirical evidence does not support a strong prior that hospital mergers improve quality. Here we discuss a few papers from the relevant literature; see Vogt & Town (2006) for a thorough review. Mutter, Romano, and Wong (this issue), examined the impact of 42 consolidations involving 136 hospitals in 16 states in 1999-2000 on 25 measures of quality using difference-in-differences models. Hospitals were categorized as acquiring institutions, target institutions, or participants in a "merger of equals." Acquiring hospitals experienced significantly improved quality in terms of abdominal aortic aneurysm mortality, iatrogenic pneumothorax, and postoperative hemorrhage or hematoma, but the quality impacts for target hospitals and "mergers of equals" were mixed.

Ho and Hamilton (2000) used difference-in-differences methods to test the impact of hospital consolidations in California between 1992 and 1995. Hospital consolidations had no impact on inpatient AMI or stroke mortality, although parameter estimates were imprecise. All three forms of consolidation (i.e., 21 mergers of independent hospitals, 54 independent hospitals acquired by a system, 65 acquisitions of one system by another) were associated with increased 90-day re-admission rates after AMI. Only the purchase of a system hospital by another system led to earlier discharge of healthy newborns. Cuellar and Gertler (2005) used 1995-2000 patient discharge data from Arizona, Florida, Massachusetts, and Wisconsin to estimate pre-post differences for facilities that reported joining a system during the study period. They found no significant changes in any of three composite measures of quality (i.e., mortality for 13 conditions and pro-cedures, utilization of 3 potentially overused procedures, and 20 potential complications of inpa-tient care) among hospitals that joined systems, except that consolidating hospitals reduced the rate of potentially overused procedures by 1.2% among managed care patients. Finally, Gowri-sankaran & Town (2003) found that competition improved quality for HMO patients, and reduced quality for Medicare patients, with the net effect being close to zero.

In addition to these empirical results, we can also take some guidance from economic theory. As discussed in Gaynor (2006), the effect of reduced competition on quality (holding the cost of producing quality constant) is theoretically ambiguous when profit-maximizing firms choose both price and quality.[14] But when prices are fixed rather than chosen by the firm, optimal quality unambiguously decreases following a competition-reducing merger; absent the ability to raise price, the only way for the firm to benefit from reduced competition is by cutting quality and thereby reducing costs. After the merger, the gain from a small reduction in quality (lower costs on retained sales) is the same as it was before, but the loss (reduced sales) is smaller because the residual demand has become less elastic. Therefore, the pre-merger level of quality can no longer be optimal and the post-merger level of quality must be lower. This result argues strongly against a U.S. hospital merger increasing optimal quality absent a change in cost, because prices are fixed under fee-for-service Medicare and Medicaid, and because these two programs (including both fee-for-service and negotiated payments) together pay for about 55% of hospital services in the U.S.[15]

Since hospital mergers are unlikely to improve quality absent a cost change, the proper focus of case-specific quality analysis is the effect of the merger on the cost of producing quality. This means that the quality analysis can be separated from the question of how the merger affects demand, and hence from the analysis of the price effects (which is convenient, as combining the analyses would be complicated). As long as the firm's optimal quality holding the cost of producing quality constant is non-increasing following the merger, a finding that the merger will not reduce those costs is sufficient (but not necessary) to show that quality will not increase as the result of the merger.

B. Sources of Quality Improvement.

Though the literature does not provide support for strong priors that a given merger is likely to improve hospital quality, it is still possible that it will do so by reducing the cost of producing quality. And there is likely a minority of mergers that can improve quality very substantially. This means that case-specific quality analysis is properly a major focus of hospital merger investigations. And as discussed above, there are well-developed methods for measuring quality, which makes such an analysis feasible.

Even in a retrospective case where direct evidence is available, the posterior estimate of the merger effect is influenced by evidence of the sort that would be used in a prospective merger case (including the question of "merger specificity"[16]). So there is value in identifying potential sources of reduced cost of providing quality and evaluating them directly. We introduce three such sources here, and defer further discussion to Section VI below. These are: (i) pre-merger clinical superiority of one hospital over another; (ii) economies of scale; and (iii) differences in resources available for investment.

i. Clinical Superiority.

One way that a merger can reduce the cost of producing quality is if one or more of the merging hospitals is operating far below its cost/quality frontier (see Pauly, 2004), and the other(s) can move it closer. That is, a merger can improve quality at one hospital if the others have superior practices or institutions that can be readily imported. If the pre-merger management of a hospital is sufficiently ineffective, the acquiring system can achieve large gains by substituting better management. See Section VI below for a discussion of how claims of clinical superiority can be evaluated. If a merger is found likely to improve clinical quality by means of exporting superior practices, this benefit would likely require geographic proximity and therefore be merger-specific, because the process of improving the inferior hospital likely requires the physical presence of personnel from the superior one.

ii. Economies of Scale.

Another way that a merger can improve clinical quality is through economies of scale in the provision of quality (which is distinct from economies of scale in producing output). There are some quality-improving pieces of equipment with high fixed costs and low marginal costs that are not worthwhile for an independent hospital or a small hospital system, but are worthwhile for a sufficiently large system.[17] A merger may put the merged entity above this threshold, resulting in additional investment in quality, or the larger of the merging entities may (with little incremental cost) be able to extend to the smaller entity the benefits of investments that have already been made. Such scale economies can be a source of improved clinical quality, but may yield only marginal benefits because investments with large benefits are likely to be made even by smaller hospitals (given that standalone hospitals face the same regulations and market expectations regarding quality as multi-hospital systems). Pure system size can have a large effect on quality only if the economies of scale are correspondingly large *and* if the interventions that provide large economies of scale are highly clinically important. There is limited evidence of such substantial economies of scale for electronic health record systems, which are costly but can yield large quality benefits due to increased data portability across sites of care and decreased incidence of medication-related errors.[18]

Another potential source of scale economies is surgical procedures that exhibit a volume-outcome relationship in which more repetition of the procedure generates better clinical outcomes for both individual surgeons and hospitals. This effect appears to be strong for high-risk, technically complex procedures, such as resection of esophageal cancer, pancreatic cancer, and aortic aneurysms, and inconsistent for lower-risk, more straightforward procedures such as "isolated" coronary bypass surgery and percutaneous coronary interventions.[19] "Learning curves" have been demonstrated for technology-dependent laparoscopic procedures, whereby operator outcomes improve with accumulated experience over time.[20] By consolidating a procedure at fewer hospitals or by sending experienced personnel from one hospital to another, a system can theoretically extend the benefits of scale enjoyed by a high-volume acquiring hospital to the acquired hospital.[21]

Other interventions that have been shown to have substantial effects on quality can be readily implemented by hospitals of any size and are thus unlikely to be related to scale.[22] Also, clinical benefits of increased scale are likely to be merger-specific only if they involve consolidation of services or sharing of personnel, as these mechanisms require geographic proximity. Some interventions, such as electronic health record systems, do not require such proximity, as the same benefits could be achieved through a merger with a geographically distant partner, and thus cannot be considered merger-specific.[23]

iii. Financial Resources.

Another possible means by which a merger can improve clinical quality is via quality-improving investments that one party to the transaction (usually the acquired hospital) was previously unable to make due to lack of financial resources. The standard theory of corporate finance suggests that firms will make those investments, and only those investments, for which the present value of the net benefits, discounted at the appropriate rate, exceeds the investment cost, regardless of the ownership of the firm. This conclusion might fail to hold if for some reason the acquiring system has a lower cost of capital than the acquired hospital. In that case, the acquired hospital would have made those investments that were worthwhile given its original cost of capital, and the acquiring system would make additional investments that would not have been worthwhile at that cost of capital, but are worthwhile given its new, lower cost. But these incremental investments are expected to be the marginal (i.e., least valuable) investments.

Any clinical quality benefit resulting from increased financial resources will not be merger-specific if there is an alternative acquirer that does not represent a competitive concern, is willing to pay a price that the acquired hospital would accept if the merger under investigation were blocked, and is willing to make similar investments. These conditions will be met if the investments are worthwhile on their own merit, but not if the willingness to make the investments, or even the willingness to undertake the merger, is dependent on the profits resulting from an anticompetitive price increase. The marginal value of incremental investments, combined with the likelihood that their benefits will not be merger-specific, suggest that enhanced financial resources are an unlikely source of significant merger benefits.

C. Health Effects of Higher Prices for Health Insurance.

Even if our analysis had found a merger-specific quality increase at the merging hospitals, the indirect effect of a price-increasing merger on health must still be considered. Higher hospital prices cause health insurance premiums to increase, which causes some people to lose or forego insurance. Town *et al.* (2006) estimated that in 2003 there were 695,000 fewer insured people in the U.S. than there would have been had there been no hospital merger activity in the 1990s. There is a substantial literature showing that lack of insurance harms health, and may be responsible for 18,000-22,000 premature deaths each year in the US,[24] although this estimate has recently been challenged by Kronick (2010). This harm would not be realized at the merging hospitals, as the people who lose their insurance would not necessarily have used the merging hospitals (or any hospital). The magnitude of this effect is difficult to quantify, as it would require estimating the insurance premium increase resulting from the hospital price increase, the number of people who would lose their insurance as a result of that premium increase, and the health harm accruing to the people who lost their insurance. But the effect is present, and it means that any measured health benefit at the merging hospitals represents an upper bound on the total beneficial effect of the merger on health. Because of the absence of demonstrable quality improvement in the ENH/HPH case, it was not necessary for us to address this question.

VI. Applicability to Prospective Merger Analysis:

This paper has focused on retrospective evaluation of the Evanston Northwestern Healthcare/Highland Park Hospital case. But the great majority of merger cases are prospective in nature, where the objective is to predict the effects of the merger, rather than to measure them after the fact. A recent example is the proposed acquisition of Prince William Hospital in Manassas,

Virginia by the Inova Health System. It is therefore worth discussing what kind of analysis of clinical quality is possible in such cases.

In section V above, we argue that hospital mergers are unlikely to improve quality absent a reduction in the cost of producing quality. Quality analysis in a prospective case should therefore focus on ways in which the merger is likely to reduce those costs, whether by means of a superior hospital exporting its knowledge and practices to an inferior one, through economies of scale, or (less likely) as a result of differences in financial resources.

Quality claims regarding clinical superiority and economies of scale can sometimes be investigated directly. The likelihood of an improvement as a result of clinical superiority is greater if there are specific quality-improving measures that have been adopted by the acquiring system and are likely to be exported following the merger. Similarly, improvements due to economies of scale are unlikely if a hospital targeted for acquisition does not actually perform the most volume-sensitive procedures, or if it has already reached a plateau on the learning curve for technology-dependent procedures.

A less direct but still valuable way to evaluate the likely quality effects of a merger is to compare their pre-merger quality levels. Large and consistent differences in these levels constitute evidence that the target hospital is under-performing and/or that the acquiring hospital is enjoying significant economies of scale relative to the acquiring system, providing potential opportunities for post-acquisition improvement.[25] These inter-hospital differences can be substantial. For example, Keroack et al. (2007) showed substantial variation in quality among academic health systems of similar size, which was linked to variation in management and organizational culture, and Jha et al. (2003) showed how the Veterans Health Administration used superior management to improve and reduce intra-system variation in clinical quality. Comparison of pre-merger quality trends may also be of some value, but can be misleading because trends may not persist, particularly if one hospital started with a much lower level of clinical performance.

Large pre-merger differences in quality levels are neither necessary nor sufficient for a merger to result in a quality increase. It is possible that a superior acquiring hospital will fail to improve an inferior one, and it is also possible that one hospital can improve another even if it is not superior. Nevertheless, pre-merger quality differences suggest that one hospital has something of value to impart to the other, absent a specific indication that it does not, for example if an acquiring hospital system had been superior to, but nevertheless failed to improve, a previously acquired hospital.

It is worth noting that in a retrospective difference-in-differences analysis, any variation across hospitals in coding practices or in patient severity that is not fully captured by risk-adjustment will not confound the analysis as long as these differences do not vary over time. In a prospective analysis, such differences in coding practices or patient severity will confound the analysis. For example, a hospital with particularly aggressive coding practices will have patients that appear sicker, and so its performance will appear better even when it really is not. So an important part of any prospective analysis is to gather as much evidence as possible regarding between-hospital variation in baseline severity of illness and coding practices.

VII. Conclusions:

There is considerable evidence that hospital mergers can cause substantial price increases.[26] These price increases can in principle be counterbalanced by pro-competitive effects, the most important of which is improved clinical quality. In this paper, we describe our analysis of the clinical quality effects of the Evanston Northwestern Healthcare/Highland Park Hospital merger.

Specifically, we use a straightforward difference-in-differences methodology to determine whether the merger resulted in improved performance on a variety of clinical outcomes measures (risk-adjusted inpatient death and complications). We find little evidence that the merger caused quality to improve at Highland Park.

On the basis of these findings, the Administrative Law Judge found "no evidence of improvement in overall quality of care relative to other hospitals."[27] We believe that our basic framework for analyzing the clinical quality effect of mergers will be applicable to future cases, including prospective ones. There are plausible mechanisms through which a merger can cause a substantial quality improvement, which means that case-specific quality analysis is important. While we take no position on how price and quality should be traded off against each other when they are in conflict, our methodological approach will characterize the magnitude of any quality effect, which can then be weighed against the predicted (or observed) price effect in the manner deemed appropriate by the decision maker.

---

[1] Dr. Haas-Wilson estimated that ENH's inpatient price increased 11.1 to 17.9 percentage points more than the price at various control groups after the merger. *See In re Evanston Northwestern Healthcare Corp.*, Dkt. No. 9315, slip op. at 35 (Aug. 6, 2007) (opinion of the Commission) *available at* http://www.ftc.gov/os/adjpro/d9315/070806opinion.pdf. Respondent's expert Dr. Jonathan Baker estimated that ENH's inpatient price increased 9 to 10 percentage points more than at his control group after the merger. *Id at* 38.

[2] Pretrial Brief of Respondent at 31, In re Evanston Northwestern Healthcare Corp., Dkt. No. 9315 (Oct. 20, 2005) (initial decision), available at http://www.ftc.gov/os/adjpro/d9315/050127resppretrialbrief.pdf; Post-Trial Brief of Respondent at 74, In re Evanston Northwestern Healthcare Corp., Dkt. No. 9315 (Oct. 20, 2005) (initial decision) available at http://www.ftc.gov/os/adjpro/d9315/050527respposttrialbrief.pdf; and Respondents' Corrected Appeal Brief at 68, In re Evanston Northwestern Healthcare Corp., Dkt. No. 9315 (Aug. 6, 2007) (opinion of the Commission), available at http://www.ftc.gov/os/adjpro/d9315/060112enhappealbriefcorrected.pdf.

[3] Additional information regarding risk-adjustment is available at the AHRQ Quality Indicators website, http://qualityindicators.ahrq.gov .

[4] See Lorence *et al.* (2003) and Santos *et al.* (2008).

[5] The other three control groups were all non-federal general acute care hospitals in the Chicago PMSA that: (i) were not involved in a merger between 1996 and 2002; (ii) had residency programs at the time of the merger; and (iii) had more than 0.25 residents and interns per staffed bed between 1998 and 2002.

[6] It is also possible that the existence of the programs at HPH improved access to those services, and thereby improved cardiac health in the broader community. We investigated this question and found no such evidence, and so we do not report those results here.

[7] See Ayanian and Weissman (2002) for an excellent summary of this literature, including description of various definitions of teaching hospitals that have been used in 20 published studies.

[8] Post-Trial Brief of Respondent, *supra* at 93; and Respondent's Corrected Appeal Brief, *supra* at 4.

[9] Post-Trial Brief of Respondent, *supra* at 83; and Respondent's Corrected Appeal Brief, *supra* at 12.

[10] See http://www.qualityforum.org/Projects/n-r/Nursing-Sensitive_Care_Initial_Measures/Nursing_Sensitive_Care__Initial_Measures.aspx

[11] Post-Trial Brief of Respondent, *supra* at 75; and Respondent's Corrected Appeal Brief, *supra* at 12.

[12] With respect to obstetric trauma, the TJC indicator includes both types of vaginal deliveries (with and without instrumentation) whereas the AHRQ indicator stratifies them to create two separate indicators. In addition, in the version of the AHRQ Quality Indicators software that we used in this analysis (Version 2.1), the numerator definition was somewhat different than that in the TJC indicator, capturing high vaginal and cervical trauma but excluding third degree perineal lacerations.

[13] Several results suggest deterioration at Evanston Hospital as well, with the notable exception of some nursing-sensitive indicators. The larger sample sizes at Evanston Hospital mean that the tests have more power, and so more results achieve statistical significance. However, it is not clear that this deterioration was a result of the merger with HPH. It is possible that the merger harmed EH through diversion of resources or lack of focus, but it is also possible that the deterioration had some other cause.

[14] Many hospitals, including ENH, are not-for-profit (NFP). There is limited evidence that NFP hospitals tend to have somewhat higher clinical quality (see Devereaux *et al.*, 2002; Eggleston *et al.*, 2008; Picone *et al.*, 2002; Shen, 2002; and Farsi, 2004), but we are aware of no direct evidence on differences between NFP and FP hospitals in their quality response to mergers. It is possible that NFP hospitals reinvest a larger fraction of the gains from competition-reducing mergers, although we are aware of no direct evidence on this question either. The quality effect of any such additional spending will depend on the pre-merger condition of the acquired hospital and on the specific investments chosen by managers of the merged entity. If the merging hospitals had adequate resources already, then the additional expenditures will likely only generate small incremental benefits (see Section V*Biii*).

[15] According to the Healthcare Cost and Utilization Project website, in 2008 Medicare and Medicaid together accounted for about 56% of hospital discharges (http://hcupnet.ahrq.gov). According to the American Hospital Association, in 2008 government payments represented about 55% of the U.S. total. (http://www.aha.org/aha/trendwatch/chartbook/2010/chart4-5.pdf)

[16] For an improvement in clinical quality to justify an otherwise anti-competitive merger, the benefit due to improved quality must outweigh (on balance, according to the decision-maker) the harm due to higher prices. But to be cognizable, a quality improvement must also be "merger specific," meaning that it would only be realized through that particular merger, and not by any other means, such as an alternative merger that does not pose competitive concerns. Since quality analysis is only relevant for mergers that are expected to cause a price increase (otherwise the quality issue will never be reached), and since price-increasing mergers usually involve hospitals that are in geographic proximity, past or future quality improvements are unlikely to qualify as merger-specific unless they require a geographically proximate merger partner. Since there was little meaningful evidence of quality improvement in the ENH/HPH case, merger specificity was not a major issue.

[17] Note that the relevant issue is the size of the *system*, not the size of the individual *hospital*. Mergers typically do not affect the size of the individual hospitals, so hospital-level economies of scale are not relevant.

[18] The role of multihospital system membership in electronic medical record adoption was explored by Li *et al.* (2008). The quality benefit of an electronic medical record with computerized physician order entry and decision support features was first demonstrated by Bates *et al.* (1998).

[19] See Halm *et al.* (2002), Killeen *et al.* (2005), and the report of the ECRI Institute (2010).

[20] See Moore & Bennett (1995) and Watson *et al.* (1996).

[21] It is also possible that the acquiring system may find it impossible to transfer its scale economies to an acquired hospital. For example, if local factors preclude shutting down a low-volume but technically complex service, or if transferring personnel across facilities is not feasible, then quality may not improve post-merger at the acquired hospital. Therefore, it cannot be assumed that any merger will lead to economies of scale related to the quality of technically complex procedures.

[22] See Provonost *et al.* (2006), Provonost *et al.* (2010), Haynes *et al.* (2009), and Weiser *et al.* (2010).

[23] It is conceivable that an electronic health record system involving geographically proximate hospitals may confer greater quality benefits than an equivalent system involving non-proximate hospitals, by allowing patients to obtain coordinated care from multiple local facilities, but this hypothesis has never been empirically tested.

[24] The estimate of 18,000 comes from the Institute of Medicine (2002); the higher estimate comes from Dorn (2008).

[25] In contrast, there is no direct link between pre-merger price level differences and the price effects of mergers, so a comparison of pre-merger price levels would not be informative.

[26] See Vogt & Town (2006), Vita & Sacher (2001), Haas-Wilson & Garmon (this issue), Thompson (this issue), and Tenn (this issue).

[27] *See In re Evanston Northwestern Healthcare Corp.*, Dkt. No. 9315, slip op. at 173 (Oct. 20, 2005) (initial decision), *available at* http://www.ftc.gov/os/adjpro/d9315/051020initialdecision.pdf.

References:

Ayanian, John Z. and Weissman, Joel S. (2002) Teaching hospitals and quality of care: a review of the literature, *Milbank Quarterly*, 80 (3), pp. 569-93.

Balan, David J. and Garmon, Christopher (2008) A critique of the "learning about demand" defense in retrospective merger cases, *American Bar Association Economics Committee Newsletter*, 8 (2), pp. 5-10.

Bates, David W. *et al.* (1998) Effect of computerized physician order entry and a team intervention on prevention of serious medication errors, *Journal of the American Medical Association*, 280 (15), pp. 1311-6.

Cuellar, Alison E. and Gertler, Paul J. (2005) How the expansion of hospital systems has affected consumers, *Health Affairs*, 24 (1), pp. 213-9.

Devereaux, PJ, Choi, PT, Lacchetti, C *et al.* (2002) A systematic review and meta-analysis of studies comparing mortality rates of private for-profit and private not-for-profit hospitals, *Canadian Medical Association Journal*, 166 (11), pp. 1399–1406.

Dorn, Stan (2008) Uninsured and dying because of it: updating the Institute of Medicine analysis on the impact of uninsurance on mortality, *Urban Institute Report*.

ECRI Institute (2010) *Hospital volume, surgeon volume and operative mortality for six procedures: a systematic review* (Washington, DC: National Quality Forum).

Eggleston, K. *et al.* (2008) Hospital ownership and quality of care: what explains the different results in the literature? *Health Economics*, 17, pp. 1345–62.

Farsi, Mehdi (2004) Changes in hospital quality after conversion in ownership status, *International Journal of Health Care Finance and Economics*, 4, pp. 211–30.

Gaynor, Martin (2006) Competition and quality in health care markets, *Foundations and Trends in Microeconomics*, 2 (6), pp. 441-508.

Gowrisankaran, Gautam and Town, Robert J. (2003) Competition, payers, and hospital quality, *Health Services Research*, 38 (6, Part 1), pp. 1403-21.

Haas-Wilson, Deborah and Garmon, Christopher (this issue) Two hospital mergers on Chicago's North Shore: a retrospective study, *International Journal of the Economics of Business*.

Halm, Ethan A., Lee, Clara and Chassin, Mark R. (2002) Is volume related to outcome in health care? A systematic review and methodologic critique of the literature, *Annals of Internal Medicine*, 137 (6), pp. 511-20.

Haynes, AB *et al.* (2009) Safe Surgery Saves Lives Study Group. A surgical safety checklist to reduce morbidity and mortality in a global population, *New England Journal of Medicine*, 360 (5), pp. 491-9.

Ho, Vivian and Hamilton, Barton H. (2000) Hospital mergers and acquisitions: does market consolidation harm patients? *Journal of Health Economics*, 19, pp. 767-791.

Institute of Medicine (2002) *Care without Coverage: Too Little, Too Late* (Washington, DC: National Academy Press), pp. 161–165, Table D.1.

Jha, Ashish K. *et al.* (2003), Effect of the transformation of the Veterans Affairs health care system on the quality of care, *New England Journal of Medicine*, 348, pp. 2218-27.

Keroack, Mark A. *et al.* (2007) Organizational factors associated with high performance in quality and safety in academic medical centers, *Academic Medicine*, 82 (12), pp. 1178-86.

Killeen, SD *et al.* (2005) Provider volume and outcomes for oncological procedures, *British Journal of Surgery*, 92 (4), pp. 389-402.

Kronick, Richard (2009) Health insurance coverage and mortality revisited, *Health Services Research*, 44 (4), pp. 1211–31.

Li, Pengxiang, Bahensky, James A., Jaana, Mirou and Ward, Marcia M. (2008) Role of multi-hospital system membership in electronic medical record adoption, *Health Care Management Review*, 33 (2), pp. 169-77.

Lorence, DP and Ibrahim, IA. (2003) Benchmarking variation in coding accuracy across the United States, *Journal of Health Care Finance*, 29 (4), pp. 29-42.

Moore, MJ and Bennett, CL (1995) The learning curve for laparoscopic cholecystectomy. The Southern Surgeons Club, *American Journal of Surgery*, 170 (1), pp. 55-9.

Mutter, Ryan L., Romano, Patrick S. and Wong, Herbert S. (this issue) What are the effects of U.S. hospital consolidations on in-hospital quality? a longitudinal analysis, *International Journal of the Economics of Business*.

Pauly, Mark V. (2004) Competition in medical services and the quality of care: concepts and history, *International Journal of Health Care Finance and Economics*, 4, pp. 113-130.

Picone, Gabriel, Chou, Shin-Yi, and Sloan, F. (2002) Are for-profit hospital conversions harmful to patients and to Medicare? *RAND Journal of Economics*, 33 (3), pp. 507-23.

Pronovost, Peter J. *et al.* (2010) Sustaining reductions in catheter related bloodstream infections in Michigan intensive care units: observational study, *British Medical Journal*, 340, pp. c309.

Pronovost, Peter *et al.* (2006) An intervention to decrease catheter-related bloodstream infections in the ICU, *New England Journal of Medicine*, 355 (26), pp. 2725-32.

Romano, Patrick S. and Mutter, Ryan (2004) The evolving science of quality measurement for hospitals: Implications for studies of competition and consolidation, *International Journal of Health Care Finance and Economics*, 4, pp. 131-57.

Santos, Suong, Murphy, Gregory, Baxter, Kathryn and Robinson, Kerin M. (2008) Organisational factors affecting the quality of hospital clinical coding, *Health Information Management Journal*, 37 (1), pp. 25-37.

Shen, Yu-Chu (2002) The effect of hospital ownership choice on patient outcomes after treatment for acute myocardial infarction, *Journal of Health Economics*, 21 (5), pp. 901-22.

Tenn, Steven (this issue) The price effects of hospital mergers: a case study of the Sutter-Summit transaction, *International Journal of the Economics of Business*.

Thompson, Aileen (this issue) The effect of hospital mergers on inpatient prices: a case study of the New Hanover-Cape Fear transaction, *International Journal of the Economics of Business*.

Town, Robert, Wholey, Douglas, Feldman, Roger and Burns, Lawton R. (2006) The welfare consequences of hospital mergers, *NBER Working Paper #12244*.

Vita, Michael G. and Sacher, Seth (2001) The competitive effects of not-for-profit hospital mergers: a case study, *Journal of Industrial Economics*, 49 (1), pp. 63-84.

Vogt, William B. and Town, Robert (2006) How has hospital consolidation affected the price and quality of hospital care? *Robert Wood Johnson Foundation Research Synthesis Report*, 9.

Watson, David I., Baigrie, Robert J. and Jamieson, Glyn G. (1996) A learning curve for laparoscopic fundoplication. Definable, avoidable, or a waste of time? *Annals of Surgery*, 224 (2), pp. 198-203.

Weiser, Thomas G. et al. (2010) Safe Surgery Saves Lives Investigators and Study Group. Effect of a 19-item surgical safety checklist during urgent operations in a global patient population, *Annals of Surgery*, 251 (5), pp. 976-80.

Table 1: Cardiac Services

	Control Hospitals			Highland Park Hospital				Evanston Hospital			
	Pre-merger rate (%)	Post-merger rate (%)	Sample Size (pre/post)	Pre-merger rate (%)	Post-merger rate (%)	Difference-in-Differences	Sample Size (pre/post)	Pre-merger rate (%)	Post-merger rate (%)	Difference-in-Differences	Sample Size (pre/post)
Coronary Artery Bypass Graft (raw) AHRQ	4.15% (0.25%)	4.00% (0.22%)	6,379	N/A	1.55% (0.89%)	N/A	0	2.67% (0.62%)	3.71% (0.73%)	1.19% (1.01%)	673
Coronary Artery Bypass Graft (risk adjusted) AHRQ	3.90% (0.24%)	3.10% (0.19%)	7,945	N/A	1.83% (0.96%)	N/A	194	4.04% (0.76%)	4.60% (0.81%)	1.37% (1.15%)	674
Percutaneous Coronary Intervention (raw) AHRQ	1.79% (0.13%)	1.54% (0.10%)	9,715	N/A	2.15% (0.59%)	N/A	0	0.76% (0.31%)	0.69% (0.22%)	0.18% (0.41%)	792
Percutaneous Coronary Intervention (risk adjusted) AHRQ	1.34% (0.12%)	1.23% (0.09%)	16,840	N/A	1.63% (0.52%)	N/A	605	0.57% (0.27%)	1.11% (0.28%)	0.65% (0.41%)	1,448

Notes:
a. The pre-merger period was 1998-1999, and the post-merger period was 2001-2003. The merger took place in early 2000, so 2000 is excluded as a transition year.
b. See text for a description of the control group.
c. Standard errors in parentheses.
d. One, two and three stars represent statistical significance at the 10%, 5%, and 1% levels, respectively.
e. "AHRQ" denotes a quality measure employed by the Agency for Healthcare Research and Quality.
f. Highland Park Hospital did not perform coronary artery bypass grafts or percutaneous coronary interventions prior to the merger.

Table 2: Advantages of Teachng Hospitals

	Control Hospitals			Highland Park Hospital				Evanston Hospital			
	Pre-merger rate (%)	Post-merger rate (%)	Sample Size (pre/post)	Pre-merger rate (%)	Post-merger rate (%)	Difference-in-Differences	Sample Size (pre/post)	Pre-merger rate (%)	Post-merger rate (%)	Difference-in-Differences	Sample Size (pre/post)
Acute Myocardial Infarction (raw) AHRQ	9.44% (0.36%)	7.42% (0.26%)	6,726	12.99% (2.53%)	7.76% (1.05%)	-3.21% (2.77%)	177	6.96% (0.87%)	8.27% (0.78%)	3.33%*** (1.24%)	862
Acute Myocardial Infarction (risk-adjusted) AHRQ	10.09% (0.37%)	8.21% (0.27%)	10,415	9.31% (2.18%)	9.65% (1.16%)	2.22% (2.52%)	644	5.68% (0.79%)	8.27% (0.78%)	4.46%*** (1.20%)	1,258
Acute Myocardial Infarction (raw) TJC	9.86% (0.40%)	7.57% (0.28%)	5,644	12.79% (2.58%)	8.77% (1.21%)	-1.73% (2.89%)	168	6.85% (0.90%)	7.56% (0.77%)	3.01%** (1.28%)	795
Acute Myocardial Infarction (risk-adjusted) TJC	10.54% (0.41%)	9.02% (0.30%)	8,916	16.52% (2.87%)	11.51% (1.37%)	-3.48% (3.22%)	545	15.26% (1.28%)	13.15% (0.98%)	-0.59% (1.69%)	1,179
Congestive Heart failure mortality (raw) AHRQ	4.13% (0.18%)	3.79% (0.13%)	11,828	5.03% (1.12%)	2.56% (0.70%)	-2.12% (1.34%)	378	4.62% (0.66%)	3.74% (0.53%)	-0.53% (0.87%)	1,018
Congestive Heart failure mortality (risk-adjusted) AHRQ	4.35% (0.19%)	3.33% (0.13%)	20,043	5.02% (1.12%)	2.39% (0.68%)	-1.60% (1.33%)	508	4.65% (0.66%)	3.44% (0.51%)	-0.19% (0.86%)	1,283
Pneumonia mortality (raw) AHRQ	9.24% (0.25%)	8.18% (0.20%)	13,827	9.33% (1.21%)	9.19% (0.97%)	0.93% (1.58%)	579	7.58% (0.73%)	9.77% (0.76%)	3.24%*** (1.10%)	1,306
Pneumonia mortality (risk-adjusted) AHRQ	8.83% (0.24%)	6.72% (0.19%)	17,997	10.16% (1.26%)	8.34% (0.93%)	0.30% (1.59%)	881	8.67% (0.78%)	9.69% (0.75%)	3.14%*** (1.13%)	1,546
Stroke mortality (raw) AHRQ	10.66% (0.39%)	10.83% (0.31%)	6,284	10.63% (2.14%)	12.14% (1.95%)	1.34% (2.94%)	207	7.00% (1.09%)	11.71% (1.12%)	4.54%*** (1.65%)	543
Stroke mortality (risk-adjusted) AHRQ	10.53% (0.39%)	9.42% (0.29%)	10,033	10.33% (2.12%)	11.65% (1.92%)	2.42% (2.90%)	280	7.14% (1.11%)	10.97% (1.09%)	4.94%*** (1.63%)	820

Notes:
a. The pre-merger period was 1998-1999, and the post-merger period was 2001-2003. The merger took place in early 2000, so 2000 is excluded as a transition year.
b. See text for a description of the control group.
c. Standard errors in parentheses.
d. One, two and three stars represent statistical significance at the 10%, 5%, and 1% levels, respectively.
e. "AHRQ" denotes a quality measure employed by the Agency for Healthcare Research and Quality. "TJC" denotes a measure employed by The Joint Commission.

Table 3: Nursing-Sensitive Indicators

	Control Hospitals			Highland Park Hospital				Evanston Hospital			
	Pre-merger rate (%)	Post-merger rate (%)	Sample Size (pre/post)	Pre-merger rate (%)	Post-merger rate (%)	Difference-in-Differences	Sample Size (pre/post)	Pre-merger rate (%)	Post-merger rate (%)	Difference-in-Differences	Sample Size (pre/post)
Decubitis Ulcers (raw) AHRQ	2.02% (0.04%)	2.31% (0.03%)	130,755	1.63% (0.21%)	1.59% (0.17%)	-0.33% (0.27%)	3,622	1.89% (0.13%)	1.59% (0.11%)	-0.59%*** (0.18%)	10,396
Decubitis Ulcers (risk adjusted) AHRQ	2.22% (0.04%)	2.39% (0.03%)	200,313	1.89% (0.23%)	1.31% (0.15%)	-0.76%*** (0.28%)	5,677	1.83% (0.13%)	1.45% (0.10%)	-0.56%*** (0.17%)	13,879
Failure to Rescue (raw) AHRQ	12.21% (0.27%)	11.03% (0.19%)	14,533	9.82% (1.99%)	9.23% (1.28%)	0.59% (2.39%)	224	11.40% (1.22%)	7.53% (0.72%)	-2.70%* (1.45%)	684
Failure to Rescue (risk adjusted) AHRQ	11.41% (0.26%)	9.81% (0.18%)	27,705	9.79% (1.99%)	5.45% (1.01%)	-2.74% (2.25%)	509	8.25% (1.05%)	5.19% (0.60%)	-1.46% (1.25%)	1,355
Selected Infections Due to Medical Care (raw) AHRQ	0.26% (0.01%)	0.29% (0.01%)	356,759	0.08% (0.03%)	0.11% (0.02%)	0.00% (0.04%)	12,523	0.12% (0.02%)	0.10% (0.01%)	-0.05%** (0.03%)	33,816
Selected Infections Due to Medical Care (risk adjusted) AHRQ	0.25% (0.01%)	0.21% (0.01%)	578,193	0.13% (0.03%)	0.08% (0.02%)	-0.01% (0.04%)	20,077	0.15% (0.02%)	0.06% (0.01%)	-0.05%** (0.03%)	49,341
Post-Operative Hip Fracture (raw) AHRQ	0.11% (0.01%)	0.07% (0.01%)	75,823	0.11% (0.08%)	0.19% (0.07%)	0.12% (0.11%)	1,818	0.03% (0.01%)	0.04% (0.02%)	0.05% (0.03%)	6,753
Post-Operative Hip Fracture (risk adjusted) AHRQ	0.12% (0.01%)	0.01% (0.00%)	127,334	0.10% (0.07%)	0.10% (0.05%)	0.10% (0.09%)	3,698	0.03% (0.02%)	0.02% (0.01%)	0.09%*** (0.03%)	11,313

Notes:
a. The pre-merger period was 1998-1999, and the post-merger period was 2001-2003. The merger took place in early 2000, so 2000 is excluded as a transition year.
b. See text for a description of the control group.
c. Standard errors in parentheses.
d. One two and three stars represent statistical significance at the 10%, 5%, and 1% levels, respectively.
e. "AHRQ" denotes a quality measure employed by the Agency for Healthcare Research and Quality.

Table 4: Obstetrics

	Control Hospitals			Highland Park Hospital				Evanston Hospital			
	Pre-merger rate (%)	Post-merger rate (%)	Sample Size (pre/post)	Pre-merger rate (%)	Post-merger rate (%)	Difference-in-Differences	Sample Size (pre/post)	Pre-merger rate (%)	Post-merger rate (%)	Difference-in-Differences	Sample Size (pre/post)
Birth Trauma to Newborn Infants (raw) AHRQ	0.55% (0.03%)	0.40% (0.02%)	58,695	0.22% (0.08%)	0.40% (0.10%)	0.33%** (0.13%)	3,559	0.26% (0.06%)	0.85% (0.09%)	0.74%*** (0.11%)	7,779
Birth Trauma to Newborn Infants (risk adjusted) AHRQ	0.54% (0.03%)	0.40% (0.02%)	94,276	0.22% (0.08%)	0.40% (0.10%)	0.33%** (0.13%)	3,982	0.26% (0.06%)	0.85% (0.09%)	0.74%*** (0.11%)	11,023
Obstetric Trauma (Vaginal with Instrument) (raw) AHRQ	23.05% (0.58%)	24.01% (0.53%)	5,336	27.29% (2.11%)	31.99% (2.42%)	3.74% (3.30%)	447	27.52% (1.83%)	35.05% (1.98%)	6.58%** (2.81%)	596
Obstetric Trauma (Vaginal with Instrument) (risk adjusted) AHRQ	22.80% (0.57%)	23.76% (0.53%)	6,473	26.75% (2.09%)	31.48% (2.41%)	3.76% (3.29%)	372	27.12% (1.82%)	34.72% (1.97%)	6.64%** (2.80%)	582
Obstetric Trauma (Vaginal without Instrument) (raw) AHRQ	9.00% (0.13%)	9.92% (0.12%)	44,965	7.26% (0.51%)	9.55% (0.50%)	1.38%* (0.74%)	2,547	10.00% (0.40%)	11.43% (0.37%)	0.51% (0.57%)	5,630
Obstetric Trauma (Vaginal without Instrument) (risk adjusted) AHRQ	9.17% (0.14%)	10.16% (0.12%)	62,909	7.75% (0.53%)	10.02% (0.51%)	1.28%* (0.76%)	3,517	10.51% (0.41%)	11.98% (0.37%)	0.48% (0.58%)	7,562
Obstetric Trauma (raw) TJC	5.49% (0.11%)	6.08% (0.09%)	39,632	7.55% (0.49%)	5.83% (0.38%)	-2.32%*** (0.63%)	2,963	6.21% (0.31%)	5.10% (0.24%)	-1.70%*** (0.42%)	6,181
Obstetric Trauma (risk adjusted) TJC	4.64% (0.11%)	5.17% (0.08%)	71,437	5.97% (0.44%)	5.35% (0.36%)	-1.14%** (0.58%)	3,885	4.90% (0.27%)	4.34% (0.23%)	-1.08%*** (0.38%)	8,153
Vaginal Birth after Caesarian (raw) TJC	37.71% (0.61%)	27.16% (0.42%)	6,287	42.01% (2.43%)	19.19% (1.72%)	-12.27%*** (3.07%)	411	43.77% (1.70%)	29.86% (1.29%)	-3.36% (2.26%)	847
Vaginal Birth after Caesarian (risk-adjusted) TJC	21.05% (0.51%)	21.29% (0.38%)	11,427	22.47% (2.06%)	22.95% (1.84%)	0.24% (2.83%)	522	21.41% (1.41%)	21.86% (1.17%)	0.20% (1.94%)	1,254
Neonatal Mortality (raw) TJC	1.08% (0.04%)	0.80% (0.03%)	53,739	0.00% (0.00%)	0.12% (0.05%)	0.39%*** (0.07%)	3,798	0.47% (0.07%)	0.51% (0.07%)	0.32%*** (0.11%)	8,617
Neonatal Mortality (risk-adjusted) TJC	1.09% (0.04%)	0.85% (0.03%)	108,588	0.28% (0.09%)	0.16% (0.06%)	0.12% (0.12%)	4,211	0.74% (0.09%)	0.82% (0.08%)	0.32%** (0.13%)	11,911

Notes:
a. The pre-merger period was 1998-1999, and the post-merger period was 2001-2003. The merger took place in early 2000, so 2000 is excluded as a transition year.
b. See text for a description of the control group.
c. Standard errors in parentheses.
d. One two and three stars represent statistical significance at the 10%, 5%, and 1% levels, respectively.
e. "AHRQ" denotes a quality measure employed by the Agency for Healthcare Research and Quality. "TJC" denotes a measure employed by The Joint Commission.

www.ingramcontent.com/pod-product-compliance
Lightning Source LLC
Chambersburg PA
CBHW080757290526
45790CB00008B/3477